Cat's Cry Syndrome
FAQs

Chapter List:

Book Introduction:

Welcome to "Whispers of Innocence: Understanding Cri-du-chat Syndrome in Cats." In this heartfelt journey, we delve into the world of cats living with Cri-du-chat syndrome, a rare genetic disorder. Prepare to be captivated by their stories, their triumphs, and the bond they share with their devoted owners.

With emotional honesty and compassion, this book seeks to educate and inspire, shedding light on the challenges faced by these extraordinary feline companions. By delving into the depths of their unique experiences, we hope to dispel misconceptions and cultivate understanding.

Chapter 1: The Silent Cry

Within the harmonious purrs and gentle meows lies a cry that remains unheard. Chapter 1 delves into the enigmatic world of Cri-du-chat syndrome, where the voice of these extraordinary cats remains muted. We unravel the history of the syndrome, tracing its origins and the discovery that forever changed the lives of affected cats and their human counterparts.

This chapter introduces you to the heartwarming individuals who embarked on this journey with their Cri-du-chat feline companions. Through their unwavering love and determination, they have become the advocates and champions of these cats, lending them a voice that resonates across the globe.

With vivid descriptions and poignant anecdotes, Chapter 1 serves as a gateway into the emotional landscape of Cri-du-chat syndrome. Prepare to be moved as you encounter the unique challenges faced by these cats and the incredible resilience they exhibit in the face of adversity.

As you immerse yourself in their stories, you'll witness the transformative power of love and compassion. Together, let us embark on this expedition of understanding, empathy, and the celebration of innocence in the face of extraordinary circumstances.

Chapter 2: Unveiling the Mystery

[]

Chapter 2: Unveiling the Mystery

In the quiet corners of their lives, Cri-du-chat

cats hold secrets that yearn to be unraveled. Chapter 2 takes us on a profound journey of discovery as we delve deeper into the mysteries surrounding this enigmatic syndrome.

With bated breath, we explore the intricate workings of the genetic landscape, seeking answers to the questions that dance within our hearts. We encounter the scientists and researchers who tirelessly dedicate their lives to unraveling the complexities of Cri-du-chat syndrome. Their unwavering determination and relentless pursuit of knowledge ignite a flicker of hope for a brighter future.

Through the power of storytelling, we bear witness to the personal accounts of families whose lives have been forever touched by Cri-du-chat cats. Their narratives unfold like delicate petals, exposing both the joys and hardships they encounter along their path. Emotions swell as we experience their vulnerability, resilience, and unwavering love for their furry companions.

In Chapter 2, we traverse the landscapes of uncertainty and curiosity, guided by the light of understanding. We embark on a quest for knowledge, eager to uncover the intricate tapestry of genes and

<u>chromosomes that shape the lives of these extraordinary cats.</u>

As the layers of mystery gradually peel away, we find solace in the embrace of a supportive community that rallies together, united by a common cause. The emotional tone of this chapter resonates with a blend of awe, fascination, and empathy as we witness the determination of these families and researchers to shed light on the hidden recesses of Cri-du-chat syndrome.

With each turn of the page, we inch closer to unraveling the secrets that lie within the genetic code of these remarkable cats. Brace yourself for a journey that will stir your emotions, leaving you enlightened and inspired by the resilience of these feline warriors and the unwavering love that surrounds them.

Chapter 3: The Genetic Landscape
[]

Chapter 3: The Genetic Landscape

In the intricate tapestry of life, every thread has a purpose, and within the genetic landscape of Cri-du-chat syndrome, lies a story waiting to be unveiled. Chapter 3 carries us into the

<u>depths of this intricate web, where the building blocks of existence shape the lives of these extraordinary cats.</u>

With a tender touch, we trace the pathways of genes and chromosomes, navigating the complex terrain of genetic mutations. Through heartfelt narratives and expert insights, we delve into the scientific realm, seeking to grasp the profound impact these alterations have on the lives of Cri-du-chat cats.

As we embark on this emotional exploration, we encounter the researchers and geneticists whose tireless efforts illuminate the path forward. Their eyes alight with passion, they guide us through the labyrinthine intricacies of DNA, unraveling the mysteries that have long confounded us.

Within the DNA strands of these unique feline companions, we discover the echoes of resilience and fragility, painted in hues of hope and determination. The emotional tone of this chapter resonates with a deep sense of empathy, as we witness the intricate dance between genetics and destiny.

Alongside the scientific revelations, we bear witness to the personal stories of families whose lives have been interwoven with Cri-du-chat cats. Their journeys navigate the peaks and valleys of joy and heartache, forever shaped by the intricate genetic landscape that binds them.

As the chapter unfolds, we come to understand that within the genetic code lies not only the blueprint of a syndrome but also the essence of resilience and love. The emotional depth of these stories beckons us to empathize, to connect, and to cherish the uniqueness that lies within each cat affected by Cri-du-chat syndrome.

With each word penned, our hearts open wider, embracing the emotional complexity of this genetic landscape. Prepare to be moved, inspired, and forever changed by the delicate balance between nature and nurture that shapes the lives of these extraordinary cats.

Chapter 4: Early Signs and Diagnosis

[]

Chapter 4: Early Signs and Diagnosis

In the realm of uncertainty, a glimmer of awareness emerges, guiding us toward a path of early detection and understanding. Chapter 4 invites us to explore the delicate nuances of Cri-du-chat syndrome, as we navigate the landscape of early signs and diagnosis.

With trembling hearts and attentive eyes, we bear witness to the subtle cues that whisper of an extraordinary journey unfolding. It is here, in the realm of the first tender moments, that the footprints of Cri-du-chat begin to emerge, painting a picture that demands our attention and compassion.

In this emotional chapter, we encounter the devoted caregivers and vigilant cat owners who possess an intuitive understanding of their feline companions. Their tales are etched with vulnerability and courage, as they recount the moments when they first noticed the distinctive signs that heralded the presence of Cri-du-chat syndrome.

Through their eyes, we glimpse the mixture of emotions that swirl within their hearts - fear, confusion, and an unwavering love that propels them forward. With empathy as our guide, we step into their shoes, feeling the weight of each decision they face on their journey towards diagnosis and understanding.

As the chapter unfolds, we are immersed in the stories of the medical professionals who play a pivotal role in unraveling the mysteries of Cri-du-chat syndrome. Their expertise and compassionate care become beacons of hope, as they navigate the delicate process of diagnosis, offering solace and guidance to families and their beloved feline companions.

The emotional tone of this chapter resonates with tenderness, empathy, and a deep desire to shed light on the early stages of the Cri-du-chat journey. It serves as a reminder that within the uncertainty lies an opportunity for compassion and growth, as we come together to support one another on this path of discovery.

With every word written, we honor the resilience of those who recognize the signs, the courage of those who seek answers, and the profound love that binds them all. Brace yourself for a chapter that will touch your soul, leaving you with a heightened awareness and a renewed commitment to understanding the intricacies of Cri-du-chat syndrome.

Chapter 5: Navigating Medical Challenges

[]

Chapter 5: Navigating Medical Challenges

Within the labyrinth of medical challenges, a symphony of strength and resilience plays out, as families and their Cri-du-chat feline companions embark on a journey unlike any other. Chapter 5 invites us to witness their unwavering determination and the profound emotional depth that accompanies

their quest for medical care and support.

In this chapter, we step into the shoes of these courageous souls, their hearts intertwined with hope and the resolute spirit that propels them forward. We witness the countless visits to veterinary clinics and hospitals, where compassion and expertise intertwine, creating a safe haven for both cats and their human caregivers.

Through tear-stained moments and smiles laced with bravery, we experience the raw emotions that accompany medical challenges. The emotional tone of this chapter echoes with a poignant blend of vulnerability and strength, as we explore the complexities of treatment plans, medications, and the ever-present uncertainties.

Amidst the hurdles and setbacks, we encounter the remarkable resilience of Cri-du-chat cats, whose spirits shine brightly even in the face of adversity. Their innate ability to adapt and thrive becomes a source of inspiration, reminding us of the indomitable spirit that resides within each of us.

Alongside the personal stories, we encounter the dedicated medical professionals who become beacons of hope, guiding families through the maze of treatment options and offering solace during difficult times. Their expertise and compassionate care become a lifeline, instilling confidence and fostering a sense of empowerment.

As the chapter unfolds, we witness the transformation that occurs within the hearts of these families. Fear and uncertainty gradually give way to resilience and determination, as they navigate the intricacies of medical challenges with unwavering love and support.

With every page turned, we are reminded of the immense strength that lies within the human spirit and the extraordinary bond between humans and their feline companions. Brace yourself for a chapter that will tug at your heartstrings, leaving you in awe of the resilience and unwavering love that permeate the journey of navigating medical challenges in Cri-du-chat syndrome.

Chapter 6: Emotional Support for Cat Owners

[]

Chapter 6: Emotional Support for Cat Owners

In the depths of their hearts, cat owners cradle a sea of emotions as they navigate the complexities of life with a Cri-du-chat feline companion. Chapter 6 extends a tender hand, offering a lifeline of understanding and emotional support to those who embark on

this extraordinary journey.

Within the pages of this chapter, we dive into the often unspoken realm of emotions, where vulnerability and resilience coexist in a delicate dance. We bear witness to the range of feelings that ripple through the hearts of cat owners - from profound love and joy to moments of doubt, fear, and even grief.

The emotional tone of this chapter resonates with compassion, empathy, and a profound understanding of the emotional roller coaster that accompanies the role of a caregiver. We explore the depths of their experiences, acknowledging the weight they carry and the strength they summon each day.

Through heartfelt narratives and shared experiences, we create a tapestry of connection, assuring cat owners that they are not alone in their journey. We offer guidance and validation, nurturing the seeds of self-care and compassion that need to be cultivated in order to support both themselves and their beloved feline companions.

This chapter introduces a spectrum of resources and strategies designed to provide emotional support. From support groups and online communities to therapy and self-care practices, we explore the avenues through which cat owners can find solace, understanding, and a sense of belonging.

As the pages turn, we witness the transformative power of empathy and community, as individuals who once felt isolated discover the strength that comes from shared experiences. We encourage open conversations and the cultivation of emotional resilience, empowering cat owners to navigate the complexities of their own emotions while providing the unwavering love and support their furry companions need.

Within the embrace of this chapter, we create a safe space where tears can be shed, fears can be expressed, and moments of joy can be celebrated. Together, we embark on a journey of healing and growth, reminding cat owners that their emotions matter, their experiences are valid, and they are deserving of the same compassion they shower upon their beloved Cri-du-chat cats.

Chapter 7: A Day in the Life of a Cri-du-chat Cat

[]

Chapter 7: A Day in the Life of a Cri-du-chat Cat

Within the rhythm of each passing day, a symphony of love, resilience, and extraordinary moments unfolds in the lives of Cri-du-chat cats. Chapter 7 invites us to step into their world, where the ordinary becomes extraordinary and every

meow carries a story waiting to be heard.

With tender eyes and hearts filled with empathy, we witness the unique experiences that shape the daily lives of these remarkable feline companions. From the moment they awaken to the world until they surrender to slumber, we walk alongside them, sharing in their joys, challenges, and the unwavering love they inspire.

In this chapter, emotions intertwine like delicate melodies, painting a vivid portrait of the indomitable spirit that resides within each Cri-du-chat cat. We witness their determination as they navigate through the intricacies of daily routines, embracing life with a fierce spirit that refuses to be defined by their syndrome.

Through the eyes of devoted caregivers, we glimpse the depth of their compassion and the lengths they go to ensure their feline companions thrive. We encounter the small triumphs and the poignant moments that highlight the profound bond between human and cat, illuminating the power of love and understanding.

The emotional tone of this chapter resonates with a delicate blend of awe, tenderness, and gratitude as we witness the magic that unfolds in the everyday lives of Cri-du-chat cats. We explore their unique personalities, quirks, and the unexpected ways they touch the hearts of those around them.

Through heartwarming anecdotes and vivid descriptions, we step into their paws, experiencing the world from their perspective. We become enchanted by the simple pleasures they savor, the games they play, and the comforting presence they bring to their human companions.

As this chapter unfolds, we are reminded that each day holds the potential for profound connection and unexpected moments of joy. In the face of challenges, these extraordinary cats embody resilience, teaching us valuable lessons about perseverance and embracing the beauty that resides in every meow.

With every turn of the page, we celebrate the unique lives of Cri-du-chat cats, cherishing the invaluable lessons they impart and the profound impact they have on the hearts of those who are fortunate enough to share their journey.

Chapter 8: Creating an Enriching Environment

[]

Chapter 8: Creating an Enriching Environment

**In the realm of compassion and creativity, a tapestry of love and care is woven to create an enriching environment for Cri-du-chat cats. Chapter 8 invites us to embark on

a journey of transformation, where the physical spaces and emotional landscapes intertwine to nurture the well-being of these extraordinary feline companions.

With gentle hands and open hearts, we explore the art of crafting an environment that caters to the unique needs of Cri-du-chat cats. The emotional tone of this chapter resonates with a deep sense of empathy, as we recognize the power of our surroundings in shaping their experiences and enhancing their quality of life.

Through insightful narratives and expert advice, we delve into the realm of sensory stimulation, understanding the profound impact that sights, sounds, textures, and scents can have on the daily lives of these remarkable cats. We learn to see the world through their eyes, honoring their heightened sensitivity and designing spaces that offer comfort, safety, and moments of joy.

Within the pages of this chapter, we encounter devoted caregivers who pour their hearts into creating environments that inspire and engage. Their creativity knows no bounds as they fashion enriching experiences through interactive toys, sensory gardens, and cozy retreats that provide solace and moments of exploration.

As we delve deeper into the art of creating an enriching environment, we embrace the principles of adaptability and flexibility, recognizing that the needs of Cri-du-chat cats may evolve over time. We encourage the practice of mindful observation and a deep understanding of their individual preferences, allowing us to continuously refine and tailor their surroundings.

The emotional tone of this chapter is one of hope and dedication as we witness the transformative power of a nurturing environment. We celebrate the caregivers who go above and beyond to create spaces that foster growth, stimulation, and a sense of belonging for their feline companions.

With each turn of the page, we are inspired to unleash our own creativity and embrace the endless possibilities that exist within the realms of design and emotional support. Together, we embark on a journey of transformation, where love, ingenuity, and unwavering dedication converge to create an enriching environment that enhances the lives of Cri-du-chat cats.

Chapter 9: Celebrating Milestones and Victories
[]

Chapter 9: Celebrating Milestones and Victories

In the tapestry of life, moments of triumph and celebration weave

<u>together to form a vibrant mosaic of joy and resilience. Chapter 9 beckons us to embrace the spirit of gratitude as we bear witness to the remarkable milestones and victories achieved by Cri-du-chat cats and their devoted caregivers.</u>

Within the emotional landscape of this chapter, we embark on a journey of reflection and celebration, honoring the small triumphs and monumental achievements that mark the path of these extraordinary feline companions. Each step forward becomes a testament to the indomitable spirit that resides within them, defying the limitations imposed by Cri-du-chat syndrome.

Through tear-filled eyes and hearts bursting with pride, we share in the joy of those who have witnessed their beloved cats reach new heights. From the first tentative steps taken, the moments of communication and connection, to the milestones of independence and resilience, we celebrate the sheer determination and unwavering love that make each victory so profound.

The emotional tone of this chapter resonates with a profound sense of gratitude and reverence as we acknowledge the incredible strength and resilience displayed by Cri-du-chat cats and their caregivers. We witness the emotional depth of these milestones, understanding the countless hours of love, patience, and unwavering support that pave the way for these triumphs.

With heartfelt narratives and shared experiences, we create a tapestry of celebration, illuminating the remarkable journeys that unfold within the lives of these exceptional cats. We recognize the courage and unwavering dedication of the caregivers who champion their feline companions, providing the love and support necessary to overcome obstacles and achieve extraordinary milestones.

As the chapter unfolds, we invite you to embrace the power of celebration, honoring the victories that may seem small to some but hold immeasurable significance within the context of Cri-du-chat syndrome. We celebrate the resilience of these cats, the unwavering love of their caregivers, and the profound impact they have on our lives.

With each page turned, our hearts fill with gratitude for the lessons of perseverance and the beauty of resilience that Cri-du-chat cats impart. Join us in celebrating these milestones and victories, for within them lies the undeniable proof that love knows no bounds and the human spirit is capable of remarkable feats.

Chapter 10: The Power of Connection and Community

[]

Chapter 10: The Power of Connection and Community

In the tapestry of human existence, there exists a thread that binds us together—a thread woven from the power of connection and the resilience of community. Chapter 10 invites us to embark on a journey that celebrates the profound impact of support networks, embracing the transformative nature of unity in the lives of Cri-du-chat cats and their caregivers.

Within the emotional depths of this chapter, we bear witness to the awe-inspiring strength that emerges when individuals come together, united by a shared purpose and a common bond. We explore the emotional landscape where compassion, understanding, and empathy intertwine, forging connections that transcend distance and time.

With tender hearts and open minds, we step into the world of support networks, where stories of hope and healing unfold. We encounter individuals who have walked similar paths, their hearts echoing with the same love and concern for their Cri-du-chat feline companions. In their shared experiences, we find solace, guidance, and the reassurance that we are not alone.

The emotional tone of this chapter reverberates with a sense of unity and belonging. We delve into the power of online communities, support groups, and social networks, where virtual hugs and of encouragement bridge the gaps of physical distance. These digital platforms become havens of understanding, offering a safe space to share triumphs, seek advice, and find comfort in the embrace of kindred spirits.

Through heartfelt narratives and shared experiences, we witness the transformative power of connection. We celebrate the friendships that blossom, nurtured by empathy and the shared journey of navigating Cri-du-chat syndrome. We recognize that, in the presence of others who truly understand, the weight of challenges becomes a little lighter, and the joys are multiplied.

As this chapter unfolds, we extend an invitation to embrace the beauty of community and the power of human connection. We acknowledge the profound impact that collective support has on the lives of Cri-du-chat cats and their caregivers, providing a lifeline of strength, understanding, and the reassurance that no one walks alone.

With every page turned, we celebrate the resilience of these extraordinary feline companions and the unwavering love of those who care for them. We honor the communities that emerge, empowering individuals with knowledge, compassion, and a sense of belonging. Together, we create a tapestry of hope, resilience, and the knowledge that we are stronger when we stand together.

Chapter 11: A Journey of Growth and Self-Discovery

[]

Chapter 11: A Journey of Growth and Self-Discovery

Within the intricate tapestry of life, the path of caring for a Cri-du-chat cat unveils a profound journey of growth and self-

discovery. Chapter 11 beckons us to embark on this transformative odyssey, where the challenges and triumphs become catalysts for personal evolution and a deeper understanding of ourselves.

In the emotional depths of this chapter, we navigate the winding roads of self-reflection and introspection. We explore the profound impact that caring for a Cri-du-chat cat has on our own lives, uncovering hidden reservoirs of strength, resilience, and compassion within ourselves.

With vulnerable hearts and open minds, we confront our own limitations and fears, finding the courage to step outside our comfort zones. We learn to adapt to the ever-changing landscape of challenges, discovering reservoirs of creativity and problem-solving that we never knew existed.

The emotional tone of this chapter resonates with a sense of vulnerability and empowerment. We delve into the moments of doubt and uncertainty, acknowledging that the journey of caring for a Cri-du-chat cat is not without its struggles. Yet, in these very moments, we find the seeds of growth, resilience, and an unwavering commitment to the well-being of our beloved feline companions.

Through shared stories and introspective narratives, we witness the transformative power of this journey. We celebrate the strength that emerges when we confront adversity head-on, the compassion that flourishes when we extend a helping hand, and the profound impact that Cri-du-chat cats have on our own identities.

As the chapter unfolds, we embrace the process of self-discovery and personal growth. We recognize that caring for a Cri-du-chat cat unlocks doors to new perspectives, deepens our capacity for empathy, and enriches our lives in ways we could have never imagined. We learn that the journey is not just about the cats we care for but also about the profound impact they have on shaping who we are as individuals.

With each page turned, we invite you to embark on this transformative journey of self-discovery. Embrace the challenges as opportunities for growth, find solace in the triumphs, and allow the unconditional love of your Cri-du-chat cat to illuminate the path ahead. For within this journey lies the profound realization that, in caring for another, we ultimately discover the boundless depths of our own humanity.

Chapter 12: Nurturing the Soul - Self-Care for Caregivers
[]

Chapter 12: Nurturing the Soul - Self-Care for Caregivers

In the symphony of compassion and love, the caretakers of Cri-du-chat cats often find themselves immersed in a whirlwind of selflessness and dedication. Chapter 12 invites us to pause, take a breath, and embark on a journey of self-care—a journey that honors the emotional well-being of the caregivers who give so tirelessly to their feline companions.

Within the emotional tapestry of this chapter, we explore the depths of the human spirit and the importance of nurturing our own souls. We recognize that in order to provide the best care for our Cri-du-chat cats, we must first tend to the gardens of our own hearts, replenishing our spirits and finding solace in moments of rest and rejuvenation.

With tender hearts and gentle hands, we delve into the practices of self-care, recognizing that it is not selfish but rather an act of compassion towards ourselves and those we care for. The emotional tone of this chapter resonates with a deep sense of empathy and understanding as we acknowledge the challenges and sacrifices that caregivers face on a daily basis.

Through heartfelt narratives and practical advice, we discover the power of self-care rituals that nurture the body, mind, and soul.

We explore the healing balm of restful sleep, the rejuvenating effects of mindful practices such as meditation and yoga, and the transformative power of engaging in activities that bring us joy and fulfillment.

As this chapter unfolds, we recognize that self-care is not just an indulgence but a necessary component of being a compassionate and effective caregiver. We learn to set boundaries, to ask for help when needed, and to cultivate a support network that uplifts and nourishes our spirits. We find solace in the understanding that our own well-being is intrinsically connected to the well-being of our Cri-du-chat cats.

With each page turned, we invite you to embark on a journey of self-discovery and self-care. Embrace the practices that replenish your soul, that restore your energy, and that remind you of the beautiful person you are, beyond the role of a caregiver. For within the depths of your own self-care, you will find the reservoirs of strength, compassion, and love that will sustain you on this remarkable journey.

Chapter 13: Embracing Moments of Wonder and Joy

[]

Chapter 13: Embracing Moments of Wonder and Joy

In the tapestry of life, amidst the challenges and triumphs, there are precious moments of wonder and joy that illuminate our path. Chapter 13 invites us to open our hearts and embrace these moments, for within them lies the essence of pure magic and the unyielding spirit of Cri-du-chat cats.

Within the emotional depths of this chapter, we embark on a journey that celebrates the small miracles and everyday joys that enrich our lives as caregivers. We witness the profound impact that Cri-du-chat cats have on our capacity for awe, filling our hearts with a sense of wonder and gratitude.

With eyes wide open and hearts brimming with anticipation, we discover that joy can be found in the simplest of momentsâ€"the gentle purr of contentment, the playful swat of a paw, or the precious sound of a heartfelt meow. We learn to savor these fleeting moments, allowing them to etch themselves upon the canvas of our memories.

The emotional tone of this chapter resonates with a childlike wonder and an unwavering sense of gratitude. We explore the transformative power of presence, immersing ourselves fully in the present moment, and finding solace in the beauty that unfolds before us. We recognize that in these moments of joy, we are reminded of the incredible resilience and zest for life that Cri-du-chat cats possess.

Through heartfelt narratives and shared experiences, we bear witness to the extraordinary connections that form between caregivers and their feline companions. We celebrate the laughter that bubbles forth, the tears of overwhelming love, and the boundless joy that arises from the unbreakable bond we share.

As the chapter unfolds, we invite you to embrace the wonder and joy that is woven into the fabric of caregiving. Treasure the moments of connection, the unexpected surprises, and the profound lessons that Cri-du-chat cats impart. Find solace in the knowledge that, despite the challenges, the journey is also one of immeasurable beauty and love.

With each page turned, we celebrate the magic that resides within the everyday. We honor the resilience and joy that Cri-du-chat cats bring into our lives, and we cherish the moments that remind us of the preciousness of our shared journey. Together, let us embrace the wonder and joy that exists within the tapestry of caregiving.

Chapter 14: The Legacy of Love and Compassion

[]

Chapter 14: The Legacy of Love and Compassion

In the tapestry of existence, there are stories that transcend time, leaving an indelible mark upon the hearts of those who bear witness. Chapter 14 invites us to explore the legacy of love and compassion that Cri-du-chat cats and their caregivers leave behind—a legacy that echoes through the ages and touches the lives of countless souls.

Within the emotional depths of this chapter, we delve into the profound impact that love and compassion have on shaping the world around us. We bear witness to the immeasurable ripple effects of a single act of kindness, as it reverberates through the lives of both humans and feline companions alike.

With hearts overflowing with love, we recognize the power of our own actions and the immense influence we have on the lives of others. We understand that the care and compassion we extend to our Cri-du-chat cats creates a legacy of empathy, resilience, and unwavering devotionâ€"a legacy that transcends boundaries and time itself.

The emotional tone of this chapter resonates with a profound sense of gratitude and humility. We honor the love that flows through our veins, breathing life into the world around us. We acknowledge the unconditional love of Cri-du-chat cats, whose spirits teach us the true meaning of compassion and acceptance.

Through heartfelt narratives and shared experiences, we witness the transformative power of love and compassion. We celebrate the profound connections that form between caregivers and their feline companions, recognizing that these bonds transcend the limitations of language and understanding. In their eyes, we glimpse the reflection of our own souls and find solace in the unspoken understanding that exists between us.

As this chapter unfolds, we invite you to reflect on the legacy you are creating through your love and compassion. Embrace the opportunity to make a difference in the life of a Cri-du-chat cat, knowing that the impact you have on their world will leave an imprint that lingers long after they have crossed the Rainbow Bridge.

With each page turned, we honor the legacy of love and compassion that Cri-du-chat cats and their caregivers embody. We recognize that the compassion we extend to these extraordinary feline companions not only transforms their lives but also shapes the very essence of our own humanity.

Chapter 15: A Forever Bond - Love Beyond

[]

Chapter 15: A Forever Bond - Love Beyond

In the tapestry of existence, there are bonds that transcend the limitations of , where love speaks volumes in the silence of a gaze, a touch, or a shared moment of understanding. Chapter 15 invites us to immerse ourselves in the profound and eternal bond that exists between caregivers and Cri-du-

chat catsâ€"a bond that defies explanation and surpasses the boundaries of language.

Within the emotional depths of this chapter, we dive into the depths of this extraordinary connection, where love becomes a language unto itself. We explore the power of presence, the beauty of empathy, and the sheer depth of devotion that exists between caregiver and feline companion.

With hearts overflowing with emotion, we recognize that the love we share with our Cri-du-chat cats transcends the spoken word. It is a love that resides in the whispers of a purr, the gentle touch of a paw, and the unwavering loyalty that surpasses any hurdle or obstacle. It is a love that speaks directly to the core of our being, reaching depths untouched by mere language.

The emotional tone of this chapter resonates with a mixture of awe, tenderness, and a profound sense of gratitude. We celebrate the moments of connection, where souls intertwine and hearts beat in harmony. We honor the strength and resilience of Cri-du-chat cats, who teach us the true meaning of unconditional love and remind us of the beauty that lies within every being.

Through heartfelt narratives and shared experiences, we witness the transformative power of this forever bond. We celebrate the laughter shared, the tears shed, and the countless memories that are etched into the fabric of our lives. We recognize that in the eyes of our beloved feline companions, we find a mirror of our own souls, reflecting back to us the essence of our deepest selves.

As this chapter unfolds, we invite you to embrace the eternal nature of this bondâ€"a bond that transcends time and space. Treasure the moments of quiet connection, the shared adventures, and the everyday miracles that unfold before your eyes. Know that the love you share with your Cri-du-chat cat is a treasure that will endure forever, even beyond the physical realm.

With each page turned, we celebrate the infinite love that exists between caregivers and their Cri-du-chat cats. We honor the depth of this bond, knowing that it is a gift that surpasses any measure of . For in this love, we discover a profound truth—that love, in its purest form, requires no language but instead speaks directly to the soul.

Epilogue: Forever in Our Hearts
[]